The Resolution Solution

Tips from Top Health and Fitness Pros

To help get you back in shape for the New Year

by Kris Crepeau

© 2013 Kris Crepeau

Disclaimer

TABLE OF CONTENTS

Introduction

It's that time of year again when we find ourselves ready to make that New Year's Resolution that we seem to make every year. We all lose our way during the Thanksgiving, Christmas, and New Year's holidays and tend to over eat a bit (or quite a bit in some cases). It's not just our diet that goes astray this time of year, we often get lax in our normal workout routine by blaming the busy time of the Holidays as our excuse. As a Personal Trainer I see it year in and year out, all of the best intentions of the New Year and a fresh start. Unfortunately, the majority of people start out strong and fade fast with their efforts in leading a more healthy and fit lifestyle.

My passion for helping people change their lives for the better led me to collaborating with some of the top health and fitness pros to provide you with their best tips, workouts, and recipes to help you get on track and stay on track for the New Year. I hope this book helps you in reaching your goals and leading a healthy lifestyle.

Bump in the Road:

I'm going to assume for the most part that those reading this book fall into the category of either having had a "bump in the road" and lost a few weeks or months of exercise or you have not exercised in years and have gained weight and need a kick in the tush. Either way, this list below is for you. For the record, a few definitions of the word "resolution" are as follows:

1. The state or quality of being resolute; firm determination.

2. A resolving to do something.

3. A course of action determined or decided on.

Definition found on wikipedia.com

A few definitions of the word "goal" are as follows:

1. the result or achievement toward which effort is directed; aim; end.

2 .the terminal point in a race.

Also: 1.target; purpose, object, objective, intent, intention. 2. finish.

Definition found on dictionary.com

Whether you call it a resolution or a goal (my personal favorite), get clear on what you really want. Make it realistic and gain some tools if you don't have them. Work towards an end result and be determined to reach the finish line.

Make sure it's something YOU have "decided" on, not your partner, not your doctor. Be firm and take action.

Get your emotions involved and imagine how you would feel when you obtain your goal. Use your imagination and ask yourself if you will look differently when you have reached your goal or resolution.

These are some of my best fitness and nutrition resolution strategies in no particular order...

• Start moving. Do something but not too much too quickly. Increase your walking. Take the stairs over the elevator when you can. Take 30 minute "get up and stretch breaks" whether at home or work.

• Make movement and light activity a part of your daily life. Put the remote across the room so you have to get up or better yet, ditch the TV and go for a walk.

• Do a combination of jumping jacks, march in place, and pushups at every commercial break when watching TV.

• Don't look at 2014 as a year of exercise and eating healthy. Start small and break it up week to week or day to day.

• Get a jump start with a simple weekly goal. Ex: "I am taking 3 bootcamp classes this week". "I'm eating breakfast every day and planning my meals".

• What kind of motivation gets you moving? Are you motivated/inspired by a future goal and pleasure? Ex: "I am working out because I want to feel better or be happier". Or are you motivated by pain? Ex: "I eat well and exercise because I don't want to get diabetes like my mother". Use whatever gets you off the couch and moving towards a healthier/fitter life. A little of both is fine.

- If you had to pick one, which would you be more willing to commit to? Eating better or exercise? Start there. Usually the two connect together in time.

- Really commit to a "sleep/wake cycle". Not many people want to exercise with only a few hours of sleep. Go to bed at regular times and do your best to wake up around the same time each day.

- Look at gaps in your schedule day to day, when you can commit to some kind of exercise, even if it's 15 minutes. Move towards 30-40 minute sessions.

- Make an appointment with yourself to workout. Write it down. Be consistent. (M - F from 8:00 - 8:45). No excuses!

- Have a plan. Be prepared. Make your workout times convenient. Pick a gym or bootcamp class close to you. Pack your gym bag the night before. Pack your lunch the night before. No excuses.

- Track your progress. Nothing keeps you motivated than seeing results. Write your workouts down. Keep track of the days you train, how you are feeling and amount lifted. Track your weight and heart rate as well.

- If it works, you see progress. Stick with it.

- Think wellness, not weight loss!

- Focus on behavioral changes rather than solely on your fitness or eating programs.

• Spend time with people who motivate and support your healthier lifestyle. Talk to the people you admire and who live the lifestyle you want and ask questions.

• Do what you enjoy not what you dislike. If you like dancing, take a Zumba class, if you like swimming take a water aerobics class. Do what you like to keep you moving. Gain the stamina and strength you need and eventually try more weight bearing activities like strength training with a trainer.

• Be accountable. Exercise with a friend who is also driven to get fitter. Join a group fitness class. A sense of community and the motivation and encouragement found there is very powerful!

• Give yourself permission to fall. Just get back up and start again.

• Give yourself one "cheat day" a week. On a heavy workout day, so your metabolism is up, enjoy that slice or two of pizza or that cup of ice cream after dinner. You worked for it!

• Have a "back up plan" should your boss tell you that you need to stay late and can't get to the gym. Have a pair of sneakers and gym pants handy and take a quick 10-15 minute workout at work.

• Try a Tabata Interval. Tabatas are 20 seconds of activity followed by 10 seconds of rest for eight rounds or 4 minutes. Try doing 3-4 Tabatas with a minute in between when getting to the gym isn't possible. Example: Pushups and Jumping Jacks. Run-in-place and crunches.

These are just a handful of what I think are useful strategies and tend to add more all the time. Feel free to try some out and see which work for you and pass them along! Have an awesome 2014. Stay fit, healthy and Thrive!

"The Bride of Frankenstein" Interval Workout

This routine includes "morphing" or combining two or three moves together to create a "Frankenstein" exercise . You can do one repetition of each exercise at at time for the required time or up to 3-5 repetitions of each exercise at a time in a flow like sequence. There are 5 circuits including two 50/10 style, one 40/20 and two final 20/10 Tabata circuits.

Warm Up 5 Minutes

Circuit One 50/10

Starburst To Alt Front Lunge

Band Reverse Fly To Face Curls

Wall Sits with Wall Slides

Band Low to High Fly To Band Elbow Behind Curls

Repeat

Circuit Two 50/10

Band Face Pulls To Alt Reverse Lunges

DB Front Raises to DB Drags

Push Ups to Diag Mt. Climbers

DB Hammer Curls To DB Triceps Kickbacks

Repeat

Circuit Three 40/20

Band Curls To Band JJ Press

DB Renegade Row To Alt Leg Raises To Close Push Ups

Band Scoops To Band Rev Fly

DB Close Grip Chest Press To DB Skull Crushers To Hip Ext

Repeat

Circuit Four 20/10

DB Deadlifts To Shrugs

DB Curl To DB Calf Raise

Repeat for a total of 8 sets

Circuit Five 20/10

DB Pec Dec to Bent Over DB Reverse Fly

Squat Hold DB Preacher Curls

Repeat for a total of 8 sets

Favorite Healthy Recipe: Sage Pork Chops

Pork chops rubbed with dried sage, salt and pepper are pan fried in butter until

golden brown then simmered in a simple beef bouillon.

Ingredients:

2 teaspoons salt

1 teaspoon dried sage

1 teaspoon ground black pepper

6 center cut bone-in pork chops

2 tablespoons butter

1 cup water

2 cubes beef bouillon

Directions:

1. Combine the salt, sage and black pepper in a small bowl and rub on both sides of the chops. Melt the butter or margarine in a large skillet over medium high heat and saute the chops for 5 minutes per side, or until well browned.

2. Meanwhile, in a separate small saucepan over high heat, combine the water and the bouillon and stir until bouillon dissolves. Add this to the chops, reduce heat to low, cover and simmer chops for 45 minutes. Serve and enjoy!

Nutritional Information:

Servings Per Recipe: 6 ,Amount Per Serving :,Calories: 159 , :, Total Fat: 7.8g , Cholesterol: 75mg , Sodium:1063mg , Total Carbs: 0.6g , Dietary Fiber: 0.1g , Protein: 20.6g

Michael Munson - Owner Thrive Fitness and Wellness, Philadelphia, PA

Staying On Track:

The biggest reason people fail to get back on track after the holidays is a lack of accountability. The best thing to keep people on track with their goals and fitness aspirations is to have accountability. Friends or coaches or someone.

It's too easy to make excuses for yourself, it needs to be a good coach. A good coach will keep you on track and check in with you. A poor coach will wait for someone to report. A good coach will seek out their client. Even a friend that will check in with the person weekly to help keep them on track is a great help.

A quick workout that can be done with little to no equipment is anything from walking for the beginners to burpees and muscle ups for the more advanced.

I recommend starting with something that matches a person's

fitness level but asks for more than their usual routine. If walking a mile is normal, jog a mile. If 20 wall pushups is normal, try kneeling pushups.

Progress is what matters most, even if slow. No workout will create an overnight dream body.

My favorite healthy recipe is just a good old fashioned Muscle Milk protein shake. It's quick, easy, and tastes great.

Matt Fellows - Iron Works Elite Fitness

You Can't do it Alone:

Reason 1: You try do to it all by yourself.

Surround yourself with people who inspire you to be more, do more, and have more," play with people better than you who inspire you to be better."

Remember, your buddy should be a positive force in your life, not a negative one. Stay away from people who drain you mentally and emotionally, even if they're willing partners.

Reason 2: Too 'big' of a goal or unrealistic.

Make small, realistic goals: Take it day by day, week by week.

Embrace the present and what can you do to make a difference in the here and now.

If you think you will lose 100 pounds in three months, this is not going to happen. You need to set a goal that is actually achievable in the timeframe you set for yourself.

Far Better to succeed at a smaller, more manageable goal than fail at a

larger, loftier one.

"New Year, New You!" LRF Workout!

Includes everything you need to build the strength, courage & confidence to make 2014 the best one yet!

Hydrate! Bring your LRF water bottle and aim to finish it by the time you are complete with workout & post stretch! You'll feel better, your skin will look better and you'll be able to fuel the body do your sweat sparkles!

Strength: you'll use your own resistance & body weight to work & build those marvelous muscles! Muscles increase metabolism, burn more calories at rest & gives you more energy! Win-win!

Balance: for life's twists & turns. Develops core strength, back, hip,knee, & ankle stability.

Endurance: by circuit training and not resting between exercises, you'll increase your heart rate which improves cardiovascular endurance as well as muscular endurance.

Flexibility: by performing a dynamic warm-up before beginning then holding your stretches post workout, you'll increase mobility in the joints, increase flexibility, and reduce stiffness, soreness & prevent injuries.

Don't forget to nourish your body with a clean source of protein within 30 minutes of your workout!

Warm up:

One set 10 exercises

30 seconds of each.

Total time 5 minutes

Jumping jacks

Squats

High kick back lunge right leg only

High kick back lunge left leg only

Burpees

Balance T right only

Balance T left only

Pushups

Plank

Back ext upper only with Y arms

1 minute each.

Beginner 1x, intermediate 2x. Advanced 3-4x

Sumo squat jumps

Burpies with push-up

Walking lunges

Diamond pushups

Front "Body rockers"abs

Post workout stretch

Hold each stretch for 15 sec

Quads

Figure 4: glutes/piriformis /hips

Hamstrings

Chest

Shoulders

Triceps

Abs

Calves

WAHOOO! High Five yourself! Less than fifteen minutes & feeling fabulous!

Favorite healthy recipe:

1 apple thinly sliced

6 to 7 cups arugula, washed and dried

1/3 cup pomegranate seeds

1/4 cup sliced almonds, toasted(preheat oven to 400 and roast for 5 mins.)

feta cheese, crumbled

Add Grilled chicken!

YUM!

Thank you!

Lisa A. Reed, MS, CSCS, USAW

Owner, Lisa Reed Fitness LLC

Plain and simple:

People fail to get back on track after the holidays because it isn't convenient. That is the straight-up truth, people are lying to you if they tell you otherwise. You fall out of the rhythm of going to the gym for a week or two and after New Year's Day roles around it just isn't convenient to drag yourself to the gym. It's not convenient to do cardio, it's not convenient to spend 45 minutes lifting weights, it's not convenient to prepare your healthy lunch the night before work.

Being healthy isn't convenient, if you make it that way. There are ways to make working out and being healthy more convenient. You have no excuses not to work out or eat healthy, if you can do it conveniently at-home.

Quick workout:

If you are crunched for time you can do what I call the "4 minute RampUp" to finish off a workout, or it could actually be your entire workout!

Basically, you pick an upper body exercise (i.e. pushups) and a lower body/cardio exercise (i.e. squats). You perform squats (can be weighted) for one minute doing as many reps as possible, then go immediately into pushups, back to squats, finishing off with pushups (each for a minute with no rest in-between). Sound easy? You'd be hard-pressed to even find a guy in your local gym that can do pushups for one minute as fast as possible. This is the best way to get a quick workout in or finish off a workout because it torches your muscles. Since there is no rest between exercises your heart rate and oxygen consumption is at a max, increasing the afterburn (keep burning calories long after your workout is over)!

It's called a "RampUp" because, if done at a very high-intensity, will keep your metabolism ramped up long after your workout is over! We all want that! If that's not enough, turn around and make it the "8 minute RampUp."

Favorite healthy recipe:

To be honest, I'm a man of simple yet nutrient-dense recipes, the ones that don't take more than 10 minutes to prepare. My favorite recipe especially for snacking is homemade hummus. There is no need to pay store prices for a small tub of hummus when you can make it the way you like it. It's amazingly easy, you just blend all the ingredients up in your food processor until they are a paste and eat with pita, veggies, wheat crackers, or whatever else you want! You can add dried tomatoes or red peppers to try different flavors! Experiment and have fun with it! Hummus in five minutes, that's pretty convenient! Here's what it takes:

1 can (15oz) garbanzo beans

1/4 cup tahini

1/4 cup lemon juice

3 tablespoons extra virgin olive oil

2 cloves of garlic

Cumin, salt, and pepper to taste

Josh Anderson, AFAA Certified Personal Fitness Trainer

Owner Always Active Athletics LLC, Jefferson City, Missouri

How to motivate yourself:

Put on your workout clothes. When it is cold or the weather is less than ideal, I often find myself procrastinating with my workouts. One way I've found of removing obstacles to winter training sessions - if I just make myself put on my workout clothes, I am way more likely to complete that workout.

When it comes to exercising, anything is better than nothing. A lot of us, when we are time crunched, tend to skip workouts entirely, instead of altering them to fit the available time. Instead of bailing on the total workout, head outside for a quick walk, or do some stretching or core work while you watch your favorite TV show.

Favorite Healthy Recipe - Fruit-Seed Energy Bars

You'll need:

9×11 glass baking dish

Mixing bowl

Dry ingredients:

1c rice crispies

1c rolled oats

1c sunflower seeds

1c pumpkin seeds

1c goji berries (these are kind of spendy, but you can sub any dried fruit or nuts)

1/2c raisins

1/2c dried cherries

1/2c unsweetened shredded coconut

Mix the dry ingredients in a big bowl.

Wet ingredients:

1c smooth almond butter

1c brown rice syrup or barley malt syrup

Heat wet ingredients over medium heat, stirring frequently, until hot and well mixed (should only take a few minutes). Then, pour over dry ingredients and mix well (work quickly because as it starts to cool, it will be harder to work with).

Pour everything into greased pan and press down evenly (spray a little cooking spray or oil on your hand to prevent sticking).

Really make sure to pack it down well, otherwise your bars might not hold together

*Optional: sprinkle the whole thing with sea salt

Chill for at least one hour (preferably 2-3) before cutting into squares. I run a butter knife around the outside of the dish and then flip it over onto a cutting board so I can cut the whole thing in squares more easily.

Georgia Gould, Cycling Olympic Medalist, U.S. National Champion, and

LUNA Pro Team athlete, Fort Collins, Colorado

Pace Yourself:

People tend to try and pick up where they left off (starting at the level they were at when exercising regularly) or start at a level that is beyond their current fitness level. They try to hit the ground running and go from 0-60 in less than 3 seconds. This causes overtraining, injury, and a sense of overwhelming failure. One typically can keep that up for the first month, but then attention wanes and illness/injury/de-motivation take hold.

I ALWAYS tell clients that they have to start with a manageable amount of time spent in the gym and take it slowly. Rome wasn't built in a day, and neither will their bodies! Instead of aiming for 5 days of working out, for 90 minutes at a time, shoot for 3 days 30 minutes the first week or two and then reassess. By making small goals, one at a time, the task of getting into shape becomes manageable and (dare I say) fun. People see results, stay healthy and get better at what they're doing, which creates more of a drive to continue. It becomes a habit that one can stick to for a much longer period of time. The longer you work at a goal, the better the outcome in the end!

Quick Workout:

CIRCUIT CITY

15-20 REPS OF EACH EXERCISE. DO EACH EXERCISE ONE AFTER THE OTHER WITHOUT REST UNTIL YOU REACH THE END. TAKE 90 SEC REST THEN REPEAT FOR A TOTAL OF3-5 ROUNDS.

REVERSE ALTERNATING LUNGES

KNEE PUSHUPS (WIDE HANDS – JUST OUTSIDE SHOULDER WIDTH)

JUMP SQUATS

KNEE PUSHUPS (NARROW HANDS – SHOULDER WIDTH)

WALL-SIT (1 MINUTE)

FLOOR/CHAIR DIPS

SIDE LUNGES

JOGGING IN PLACE (1 MINUTE)

SUPERMANS

JUMP LUNGES (EACH JUMP IS ONE REP)

Favorite healthy recipe

South-Of-The-Border Chicken & Rice Soup

A bowl of this homemade soup is a wonderful meal to enjoy during the

holidays. It's low carb and filled with protein and veggies to power your

day and curb your cravings. Best of all it's made in the slow cooker, so

preparation is quick and easy. *Servings: 8 *

Here's what you need...

- 2 organic, free range chicken breasts

- 1 (28oz) can diced, fire roasted tomatoes

- 1 (4oz) can green chiles, chopped

- 1 yellow onion, chopped

- 2 cloves garlic, minced

- 1 head cauliflower, shredded

- 32 oz organic, free range chicken broth

- 2 teaspoons ground cumin

- Dash of sea salt and pepper

- 1/4 cup fresh cilantro, chopped

- 2 avocados

- Tajin seasoning for garnish

1. Combine all of the ingredients, except the cilantro, avocado and tajin, in a slow cooker. Cover and cook on high for 3 hours.

2. Remove the chicken breasts from the slow cooker. Shred with a fork and then return to the slow cooker.

3. Garnish each bowl with a sprinkle of cilantro, a few slices of avocado and a dash of tajin. Enjoy!

Nutritional Analysis: One serving equals: 153 calories, 6g fat, 321mg

sodium, 14g carbohydrate, 7g fiber, and 10g protein.

Jennifer Searles Owner, The Works Personal Training Studio in NYC and

Team Works Figure and Bikini Team

Picking the Right Goals:

The biggest reason people fail after making a resolution to 'get in shape' or 'lose 20 pounds' is because they set the wrong goals and don't immediately see results. Choosing to increase your fitness level or shed pounds is wonderful, but it's also very vague. With a plan to 'lose 15 pounds', frustration will set in quickly because it takes a long time to lose 15 pounds. After a few weeks of not making the goal, most people give up. Similarly, stating your goal for the new year is to 'get in shape' doesn't really mean anything. What is 'in shape'? Does it mean run 5K in under 30 minutes? Be able to do 100 push-ups?

Goals need to be specific, measurable, time oriented and attainable. 'I want to lose 20 pounds' is specific, measurable and attainable, but not in a reasonable time frame. If it takes too long to see results, people quit. A goal that reads 'I want to lose two pounds per week for X number of weeks' is specific. The goal is to lose weight. It's measured by standing on a scale and attainable because losing two pounds per week is a healthy weight loss rate, but it is also time driven. You have one week to succeed for fail. It's likely that if you do fail, you'll get right back up and try the next week because you haven't had time to get frustrated. If you succeed and hit the goal, no matter how small, it's a huge accomplishment that motivates you to continue. The best way to prevent having a New Year's Resolution failure is to set reasonable, short term specific goals.

One of my favorite body weight workouts is the Deck of Cards. All you need is a set of 52 playing cards and your body. You move through the deck as fast as you can, taking the cards as they come. Each suit represents an exercise and values for the cards are as follows: Ace – 15 reps, King – 13 reps, Queen – 12 reps, Jack – 11 reps, 10-2 – face value reps. While the exercises can be anything, my favorite four are Burpees (hearts), sit-ups (diamonds), push-ups (spades) and air squats (clubs). To do the workout, simply shuffle the cards and place to stack face down within arm's reach. Flip the first card over and get going. This is a great workout to time and repeat every four to six week to gauge progress.

A great healthy recipe that I love is this Chicken, Broccoli and Quinoa Casserole. It's a healthy, tasty replacement for the carb, cheese and fat loaded Mac n Cheese.

Prep Time: 10 minutes

Cook Time: 15 minutes

Servings: 4

Difficulty (1-10): 5

Ingredients:

2 chicken breasts, thawed and cubed

1 can Campbells Healthy Choice Cream of Chicken Soup

1 cup frozen broccoli

1 cup uncooked quinoa

2 tablespoons olive oil

Salt and pepper

Instructions:

-Bring one cup of quinoa and two cups of water to a boil, adding a small amount of salt

-Simmer for 10-12 minutes or until you can see the germ separating from the seed

-Heat oven to 375

-Brown cubed chicken over medium heat with olive oil

-Completely thaw broccoli and mix with browned chicken. Using frozen that isn't thawed can make the mixture watery.

-Pour cream of chicken soup over chicken and broccoli, heat

-Mix cooked quinoa into casserole then add in chicken, soup and broccoli, stir

-Top with low fat cheese if desired, season with salt and pepper as desired

-Heat in oven for 10 minutes or until cheese in bubbling

Meredith O'Brien, MS Virginia Beach, Virginia

Consistency is Key:

Most people try to achieve their goals in unrealistic amounts of time and they are too sore to move after their first workout or they don't have goals other than the fact that they joined a gym like they said they would so, they end up not getting any results at all. I have seen this happen consistently year after year...people sign up Jan. 1 with the "this is the year I get fit....". Unfortunately, about 70% of our US adult population is now overweight or obese and working out every now and then or for the first two weeks of the year isn't going to work.

My must have's to make your resolutions work are:

1) *Set a Goal*; make it realistic and start small. For example, my clients successful goals may look like this: I want to lose weight and have more energy so, I commit to exercising every day for the next 30 days. Set yourself up for success. Unsuccessful goals may sound like this: I am going to lose 15 pounds this month, not drink alcohol, not eat out, ...you get the idea.

2) *Be Consistent*. Even the best goals and intentions may have moments where we fall short. Take the small victories. For example, if you have to work late, your kid is sick, or any other of the myriad of reasons come up that you can't do your full exercise routine then simply do one thing; 10 squats before you brush your teeth, calf raises while cooking dinner, take the stairs instead of the elevator.... These small actions will keep the momentum going and while they may not be as good as a sweat drenched post workout feeling, any activity you do is always better than none.

3) *Have fun! *Yes, I said have fun and enjoy exercise because when you like what you're doing you are far more likely to stay with it. If you don't like going to the gym then go to a park to exercise. Pick things you like to do and make sure the location is convenient to where you live or work so, that won't become a reason why you don't stay active all year long.

Here's a recipe that's tasty and good for bringing good luck in the New

Year:

Recipe - Creole-style black-eyed peas

Ingredients:

3 cups water

2 cups dried black-eyed peas

1 teaspoon low-sodium chicken-flavored bouillon granules

2 cups canned unsalted tomatoes, crushed

1 large onion, finely chopped

2 stalks celery, finely chopped

3 teaspoons minced garlic

1/2 teaspoon dry mustard

1/4 teaspoon ground ginger

1/4 teaspoon cayenne pepper

1 bay leaf

1/2 cup chopped parsley

Directions:

In a medium saucepan over high heat, add 2 cups of the water and black-eyed peas. Bring to a boil for 2 minutes, cover, remove from heat and let stand for 1 hour.

Drain the water, leaving the peas in the saucepan. Add the remaining 1 cup of water, bouillon granules, tomatoes, onion, celery, garlic,mustard, ginger, cayenne pepper and bay leaf. Stir together and bring to a boil.

Cover, reduce heat and simmer slowly for 2 hours, stirring occasionally.

Add water as necessary to keep the peas covered with liquid.

Nutritional Information per serving:

Calories 173

Total Fat 1 g

Protein 11g

Carbs 31 g

Drew O'Connell – Master Trainer, Now Body Fitness

Why People Fail:

People typically fail after the holidays because they try the one size fits all approach to getting healthy. When, in fact, we are each very different in what will make us succeed and stick to healthy habits. This 'one size fits all' approach focuses on a broad outcome (ie: lose weight, exercise more), rather than focus on individual changes that will move them towards their goal. When people can assess their goal from the perspective of what specific changes they need to make, they stay more focused on the important behaviors that need to change to achieve the goal.

For example - We all know that to lose weight one needs to cut down on calories. But the best way for each person to do this is different depending on his/her specific habits. One person may need to quit eating fast food while another may need never eat fast food, but has a bad habit of snacking after dinner adding empty calories to their daily total.

When they approach a goal based on "one size fits all" they might cut calories for a while, but when things get tough they fall back into familiar habits that sabotage their goals after the Holidays. This happens because they don't identify the specific habits that are holding them back from having long term success.

Solution

When I work with clients we make a master list of all the things they could change to achieve their goal. Then we narrow it down to the 2-3 they are willing to do consistently - day in and day out! By getting to choose what they work on it builds confidence in their ability to change and they are more willing to tackle the things they perceive to be harder to do.

So, encouraging people to identify the habits that are keeping them from achieving their goals will help them succeed at getting back into healthy habits after the Holidays. This also helps them realize bad habits they may have picked up over the holidays that need to change!

Paula Stephens, M.A., ACSM CPT

Don't Procrastinate:

Many people struggle with just getting to the gym, or taking the first action on their fitness goal. I think this comes from knowing well before January 1 that you have this goal. The problem is, if you have a goal, and you wait to take action on it, that procrastination becomes habit with your goal. When you know you have a goal, start working towards it! You don't need to wait for a calendar or a time. Take steps forward immediately. When you know in December you have a fitness goal, but you wait until January to act on, it is much harder to get started and to stay consistent, because you have already conditioned your mind to delay this goal. Don't make procrastination part of your routine. Make action your default setting.

- Quick workout that can be done with no or minimal equipment.

Not only is Barre the hottest new fitness trend, it's a great workout!

Ballerinas have been doing the same exercises for hundreds of years, because they work! Because these exercises don't require any equipment, besides your body, you can get your workout in at home or while travelling!

No excuses! You can have a great, full-body workout, wherever you are!

Things to Keep in Mind

Engage your postural muscles:

Pull your navel to your spine and drop your tailbone towards your heels.

Pull your shoulders down and back. Imagine a zipper between the two sides of your ribcage in the front, so your upper abdominals are engaged. If you have done all of this, you should feel tight, but lifted, in your core.

Moving with control means controlling even the parts of the body that are

NOT moving!

Work with resistance, not momentum:

Remember, we are doing the movement AND resisting it, to make long, lean, strong and flexible muscles. To help with that--

Use your imagination:

This engages your mind and your body. Focus on your movements, execute them with control, and you will have a more effective workout. Joseph Pilates, the creator of Pilates, used to say "It is the mind that guides the body."

He knew keeping your mind focused would lead to a deeper workout! This also increases your brain/body communication skills, which is important for motor control, injury rehabilitation.

I'm going to give you instructions and images to help you through the exercises for your glutes and arms:

Arms- Bicep Curls

Hold your arms out straight in front of your shoulders, palms up. Stand tall, stomach pulled in, shoulders down.

Imagine 100lb weights in your hands.

Keeping your elbows in line with your shoulders, bend them, so your hands come towards you.

Can you feel the weight? Feel your bicep strengthening here!

Continue pulling your lower arms up, so your elbows are at 90 degrees, with your wrists in right over your elbows.

Continuing to keep your elbows up, stomach in, shoulders down, press your hands back down to where you began.

Feel the bicep lengthen, and your tricep strengthen.

Repetitions- 3-5

Alternate Image- If the weight in the hands image isn't working for you, try this- your personal trainer, or a football player, or Arnold Schwarzenegger, is standing in front of you. He has his hands on top of yours. To pull in to 90 degrees, you must also pull his hands up. To press back down, imagine his hands on the back of yours. You must now push him away.

Glutes- Arabesque Leg Lift to the Back

Arabesque is a ballet term that means- A pose on 1 leg, with a straight leg in the air.

Set-up- Stand facing a ballet barre or chair. Only 2 fingers of each hand are on the barre/chair. It is there just to assist with balance, not to hold you up!

Begin with your right leg extended behind you, with your toes on the floor.

Draw your navel into your spine to support your back. This is very important to prevent low back strain in this exercise! You'll know you are doing this correctly if you keep your body upright, not dropped over towards the barre. If you feel a strain in your low back, engage and lift your abdominals more.

Pull your right leg up behind you with control, taking a 4-count to reach your highest point.

Imagine there is a big rubber band around your ankles, and you are pulling it apart as you lift your leg.

Press the right leg back down to your starting position taking a 4-count to do so.

Don't let the rubber band snap in. Slowly press it closed.

Repetitions- 4 times on each leg.

Progress it- Do the exercise free standing. This increases your core work, as you have to balance. Lift the arms up and out to the sides for bonus arm work!

Nicole LaBonde - CABARRET Barre & Dance Fitness

Miami, Florida

Be Specific With Your Goals:

In my experience, the biggest reason people go off track after the New Year's is that when they set themselves up for failure by setting goals that are either too vague or too big to be tackled on their own. Some examples would be "I want to lose weight" or "I want to lose 20 pounds in a month."

The solution that has worked best in my experience is to have them define smaller goals as steps to a larger goal and to make those goals something concrete and manageable. Some examples would be to start a regular workout, get a workout or goal partner for support and accountability.

Quick workout:

1. Squats - low and slow. Inhale on the way down, exhale on the way up.

Start with a 3-5 count down and another 3-5 count coming back up. As you get stronger, up the count. 10 reps is a good place to start.

2. Wall push - one leg behind, keep the torso vertical, arms slightly bent. Pull the abs in and up, 10 toes slightly grip the floor and press and hold the press for a 5 count. Repeat 10-20 times.

3. Knee ups - Hold the palms starting waist level and alternate lifting the knees to touch the palms. Keep the body vertical and no slouching. This can be done slow to start, but to add a cardio kick, pick up the pace.

Same side hand is recommended to start, but for variety, alternate hand/knee (left hand, right knee) can be added later.

Favorite healthy recipe - Fall Kale Salad

Ingredients:

- 1 head kale, cleaned and stems removed

- 1 teaspoon sea salt

- ½ cup fruit juice sweetened cranberries

- ½ cup raw pumpkin seeds

- 1 pear, chopped with the skin on

- 1 carrot, shredded

- ½ cup olive oil

- 2 tablespoons raw apple cider vinegar

Directions:

Heat oven to 350 degrees.

Put clean kale leaves into a large bowl. Sprinkle salt on leaves and massage with hands for 2-3 minutes or until leaves begin to soften. Let kale sit while you chop and prepare other ingredients.

Spread pumpkin seeds in one layer on a large baking sheet. Place in oven and toast lightly, stirring once or twice. Seeds are done when they turn slightly brown and you just begin to smell them, about 5 minutes. Watch the seeds closely as they burn easily.

Combine kale, cranberries, pumpkin seeds, pear and carrot in large bowl. In a separate bowl, combine olive oil and apple cider vinegar. Whisk until well blended. Pour mixture over the salad and mix well.

Salad can be served immediately, but is much better after it sits for a couple of hours or even the next day. Keeps four days in the refrigerator.

Drew Vanover - Yoo's Martial Arts, Tarrytown, NY

Falling off the Wagon:

People fall off the wagon during the holidays because they're too busy celebrating the season (excess food/drink) to keep up with the active lifestyle they normally try to maintain. Here are three tips to combat this:

1) Make exercise part of your social plans. Instead of meeting for drinks before dinner, try something active like ice skating or snow shoeing instead. It's festive, it's active, and it keeps you in motion, too.

2) Leave the party early to get precious sleep. Keeping your mind and your body healthy going into the new year begins with sleep. It refreshes, re energizes, and revitalizes your body.

3) Eat healthy food before you leave to go to a party. With cookies, cakes, and alcohol on the menu, a holiday party can ruin your sleek physique. So eat food you know is good for you before going to the holiday shindig, and you'll be ahead of the curve on January 1st.

Holiday workout at home (20's)

-20 push ups

-20 sit ups

-20 crunches

-20 jumping jacks

-20 second jump rope intervals

-20 leg lifts

-20 scissor kicks

"Quick protein bowl"

Combine 1 can of tuna (water drained) with 1 cup of lowfat cottage cheese.

Fold in a handful of roasted, salted cashews. Top with fresh salsa and enjoy!

Eric "The Trainer" Fleishman, Muscle and Fitness advisor, Gold's

Gym spokesperson and Hollywood Physique Expert

Being Realistic:

Many people fail due to lack of realistic goal setting, and lack of an accountability partner. As a therapist, coach, trainer, and nutrition counselor I tell clients to set SMART goals.

Specific

Measurable

Attainable

Realistic

Time Sensitive

If they set goals in this manner, and have a professional or dependable accountability partner, success is increased.

I tell clients to put a reminder in their phone, it should go off daily.

Ideally it will off at the time of day, that they are most vulnerable. This a reminder of their Why's! Why did they set the goals, Why must they attain them.

Lastly, you can't have the same people in your life, do the same things, and think the same ways, and then expect change. New social circles, new experiences and hobbies, and allowing your thought process to be challenged are absolutely necessary.

Quick workout:

Tabata Workout: Download a Tabata App for your phone.

Set it to 20 seconds Exercise, 10 Seconds Rest, and 30 Seconds Transition.

Cycles=8 and Tabatas are 6

Squat

Pushup

Reverse Lunge

Planks

Jumping Jacks

Military Pushups alternating with Situps

Favorite healthy recipe:

Green Smoothie in Nutribullet or extraction blender:

Handful of Kale, another of Spinach (steamed in adv are preferred)

2 stalks celery, handful of baby carrots,

8oz water, 1 pack of strawberry Emergen-C,

1 cap Apple Cider Vinegar. Blend until Smooth

Add one scoop Vegetarian Protein Powder in, and blend again

Tiffany Brown MS, LPC Holistic Psychotherapist

Owner, Fit 4 Life, CEO Nikki Enterprises Inc.

Be Flexible with your Diet:

One of the biggest diet traps I see is creating "forbidden food" lists. Dieting is doomed to fail if it creates no space for flexibility. Yo-yo dieting (which typically results from extreme restriction diets, followed by binging because you can't adhere to that kind of diet for very long) can be extremely hard on your metabolism and will actually raise your body's natural set point or natural weight. The key to getting back on track after the holidays is to aim for balance! Don't set out on a super strict diet that cuts out sugar, fat and gluten all at once. Instead, try the 80/20 method - 80% healthy food (whole grains, produce, unprocessed, etc) and 20% fun food. This is much more doable, and more healthy in the longterm.

Quick workout:

Mini yoga series.

There are awesome 5-10 minute yoga sequences available on youtube for free or get a membership with yogaglo.com where you can access hundreds of classes of different lengths. You just need a quiet space and your laptop or phone. Yoga builds strength and flexibility, while also grounding and relaxing you.

Favorite healthy recipe:

My go to breakfast (or snack) is greek yogurt paired with seasonal fruit (right now, apples, persimmons, pomegranates),with homemade granola and a drizzle of honey. Delicious and nutritious!

Laina Copley - Juicy Body Love, Santa Cruz, CA

What are your expectations?:

Biggest reason people fail with weight loss post-holiday? Unrealistic expectations! Setting weight loss goals that are too fast to achieve or too difficult to maintain is a recipe for failure. Reasonable, measurable goals in an appropriate time frame will not only boost motivation but also achieve lasting results!

Quick workout:

Any exercise routine that combines cardiovascular (to boost heart rate) and strength training (to build and maintain muscle) will yield measurable results. To maximize time, move from one strength training exercise to another, rapidly. Quickening the pace will get the heart rate up. Using body weight is an excellent choice. Here's a sample workout:

-5 min jump rope

-30-45 second front plank

-10 push-ups (on the knees for an easier modification)

-30 second side plank (do both sides)

-Walking lunges, 2-4 times across the room. (Add dumbbells for extra challenge)

-10 burpees (stand, squat, kick legs out and in back to squat. Repeat)

-25 crunches

-roll over on belly-elevate arms and legs in a "Superman" pose. Hold for a five count, lower, repeat 3x.

If you have more time, you can add up to 3 additional sets of each exercise.

Stretch!!! Stretching is a part of every complete workout.

Favorite healthy recipe:

I love a hearty lean-protein, lotta-veggies soup after a winter workout. It's healthy, filling and hydrating! Make sure to choose a broth over a bisque (lower in fat.)

Dayna M. Kurtz, LMSW, CPT Manhattan, NY

Set Small, Measurable Goals:

The biggest reason I think people fail at keeping to their resolutions after the New Year, is that they are overly ambitious with their immediate goals. They soon realize that it takes too much time and effort to implement the drastic changes and get discouraged. My suggestion to them is to try making smaller, gradual changes that you will actually stick with over time and add new ones after you've given yourself a chance to create a habit. Baby step it... Meal delivery services, like Factor 75, will allow you to start eating healthy without having to learn how to grocery shop and cook healthy. It's convenient and saves time so you are more likely to stick to a routine without taking additional time away from your already hectic schedule.

Quick workout:

I prefer bodyweight workouts that can be done anytime, anywhere. Do rounds of 3 minutes, 1 minute each exercise with a 60 second break in between. An example is: squats, pushups and crunches. You can change it up with lunges, burpees and jumping jacks. There are all sorts of easy activities you can do with this schedule and by doing shorter, more intense workouts you end up burning a lot more calories than a typical jog or elliptical. It also increases your metabolism more than regular jogging or similar exercises.

Favorite healthy recipe:

Factor 75's Butternut Squash Lasagna is one of my favorite recipes because it is easy to prepare, tastes great, and can show you that eating healthy doesn't have to be miserable.

Butternut Squash Recipe

Hardware:

2" casserole dish

Large frying pan

Sauce pan

Heat resistant spatula

Knife

Cutting board

Peeler

Large metal spoon

Ladle

Latex gloves

Ingredients:

2 Large Butternut Squash

1 Large Red Onion

1 lb Ground Turkey

½ Tablespoon Powdered Sage

1 Teaspoon Granulated Garlic

Black Pepper

Pinch of Crushed Red Pepper

1 Teaspoon Fennel Seed

1 Teaspoon Kosher Salt

2 28oz Can Crushed Tomatoes

2 Cups Water

1oz Parsley

2oz Celery

1 Tablespoon Chopped Fresh Garlic

1 Cup Red Wine

1 Tablespoon Blend Oil

This is a very simple and delicious recipe that can be made at home with minimal prep time and execution. You can also use your favorite store bought tomato sauce and/or turkey sausage if you choose.

Directions:

First you will want to get your tomato sauce cooking; pick, wash and chop approx. 1 oz. of parsley. Celery should also be chopped fine (a food processer works just fine) and this should be about 2 oz., these two ingredients can be kept together on a small plate as they will go into the saucepot together.

In your saucepan on medium heat, add 1T of blend oil and then 1T of garlic chopped at this point add a pinch of crushed red pepper. Once the garlic is frying (but not browning) add your parsley and celery, stir and fry for approx 2 minutes. One cup of red wine is next and let that cook until almost dry. Add your crushed tomato and rinse out the cans with water (about 2 cups), stir to combine, season with salt and pepper to taste.

Bring up to a boil and down to a simmer for around a half an hour.

While your sauce is simmering we will make the sausage crumble, in a frying pan toast 1t of fennel seeds on low heat. When they are nicely toasted add your ground turkey, season with a teaspoon of salt, pinch of black pepper and chili flake, 1/2T of sage powder and 1teaspoon of granulated garlic. Cook over high heat stirring occasionally to create a desired crumbled texture to the meat. Reserve to the side and let cool. If using store bought sausage remove the casing and fry in the same manner.

Don't forget to stir your tomato sauce!

Peel your onion and butternut squash, julienne the onion and place in a bowl. Next peel the squash (you may want to use gloves for this) cut once where the seed pod and the neck separate. Cut these two pieces in half lengthwise, and using a spoon scrape out the seeds and strings from the seedy part of the squash (just like a pumpkin). Cut these into half-moons about ½" thick and place in a bowl then toss with 1T of blend oil and sage powder and mix until all are seasoned evenly.

By now your tomato sauce should be done and we are ready to assemble the casserole. Have your onion and sausage next to each other and the tomato sauce next to that with a ladle. Your casserole dish in the middle with the squash to the other side of the onion, sausage and sauce; this assembly line will make it easy to make our lasagna. Start with a layer of sauce on the bottom of the dish, then pick out the nice ½ moon pieces of squash and starting in the corner lay them in a shingle like pattern moving north to south until the bottom layer is formed. Then using your hands (gloves of course!) take half the sausage and sprinkle it in an even layer, followed by the onion. Ladle tomato sauce in rows over this layer approx 3 ladles. Next we want to use the thinner part of the squash from the seed pod to build the center layer of the lasagna; arrange them (a little overlap is ok) leaving as smooth of a surface as we can, then repeat our sausage and onion sprinkle and sauce layer. Finally we should have enough of the nice ½ moon pieces to form another shingle layer for the top. Cover with remaining tomato sauce carefully filling in holes and making a nice smooth layer for the presentation side.

Cover the lasagna with aluminum foil and bake in a 425 oven for approximately 2 hours (depending on your oven). Test the center with a probe (your clean knife will work just fine) when our lasagna is done the probe should slip in as if it were wet sand, a little resistance but no real pressure exerted. Let cool and cut to desired size and enjoy!

I recommend a nice bitter greens salad or sautéed greens (kale, chard, spinach, etc) and a glass of the wine that you used to make your sauce.

Nick Wernimont is an ex MMA fighter and pro athlete who recently founded Factor 75 Chicago, IL

The Larger Issue of Why We Often Fail:

I developed a performance model called "The Reflex" which I taught to the good people at Mars. The Reflex addresses the root issue of why we fail at our New Year's Resolutions - we are reflexively conditioned to do so. We are conditioned through marketing, advertising and media to give our power for change to things outside of ourselves.

Magic diets, exercises, equipment and apps. We fail because we keep everything in our heads, but change only comes when we feel like it. Yes, we know should take care of ourselves and we know should make eating properly and exercise a priority. We understand intellectually that this is the right thing to do, and yet for most of us, we don't stick with it long enough to get our results, simply because our sub-conscious mind doesn't feel like it.

The reality is that most of our decisions are made from conditioned, sub-conscious minds. You see, when our attention, what is in our head, is attached to our intention, what we feel, then the power for lasting change can occur. Until we mix what we think we should be doing with our heart and feel that we want to do it, it won't get done - period!

How to change your reflex and put this into practice.

One powerful component to The Reflex is to perform a simple writing exercise, ideally first thing each morning, before you interface with anything. With pen/pencil and paper, take about 1 minute and write down your goal and then an action step that supports that goal. Write this over and over until you fill the page. Then, get up and do it! Then "Check Your Mind" to discover how you feel. Now move on with your day.

Quick Workout:

Pushups (on knees, full, inclined on chair, desk, bench, etc)

Squat Row w/tubing (if available)

Walking lunges or jumping switch lunges

Rotating Side/Front/Side Support (planks) with or without leg raise.

Hold each position for 3-5 sec.

Sit ups. That's right, one of the functions of your rectus abdominis is to flex your ribs towards your pelvis so you can, you know - Sit Up!

Good ole' Burpees. Pushup to squat jump - repeat.

If space is available, timed 15 - 30 sec sprints

Perform as circuit, one exercise after another. Rest for 1 - 2 min between circuits or until heart rate/pulse is down around 120bpm. Repeat 2-4 times.

Favorite healthy recipe:

Salad

Sliced chicken breast or salmon

Romaine, mixed baby-kales and baby spinach

Sliced oranges, watermelon and/or pineapple

Sliced Jicama

Pine Nuts

Dressing - Honey, orange juice and balsamic vinegar

Although these may sound like odd combinations, just try it, it's awesome!

Chris Weiler - Published Author | Speaker | Trainer | Coach

Chicago, IL

4 Week Resolution Solution Total Body Workout

This workout will be performed in intervals. For example if you see the interval 50/10, you will perform each exercise at max effort for 50 seconds and then rest for 10 seconds before moving on to the next exercise. The only equipment you will need for this workout is an exercise band. Most exercises are well known and can be found on youtube if you are unsure of the movements.

The workouts are set up for Monday, Wednesday, and Friday. On Tuesday and Thursday I recommend staying active playing golf, sports, or go for a run.

Week 1 and Week 3:

Monday – Chest and Back

Circuit 1 50/10 Repeat for 2 sets

Push Up

Band Row

Burpee

Band Side Lateral Raises

Circuit 2 50/10 Repeat for 2 sets

Diamond Push Up

Band Lat Pull Down

Walking Push Up

Band Front Lateral Raises

Circuit 3 30/30

Dive Bomber Push Up

Band Bent Over Row

Band Resisted Push Up

Band Pulls

Burpee w/push up

Alternating Band Front and Side lateral raises

Circuit 4 20/10 Repeat for 2 sets

Staggered hand Push Up

Band Shoulder Press

Wide Push Up

Band Arnold Press

Wednesday - Bi's and Tri's

Circuit 1 50/10 Repeat for 2 sets

Alternating Band Curls

Band OH Tri Extensions

Hammer Curls

Band Tri Kickbacks

Circuit 2 50/10 Repeat for 2 sets

Band In/Out Curls

Diamond Push Up

Band Curl Up/Hammer Down

Chair Dips

Circuit 3 30/30

Band 21's

Band Skull Crushers

Band Iso Curls

Band Throw the bomb L Arm

Band Concentration Curls

Band Throw the bomb R Arm

Circuit 4 20/10 Repeat for 2 sets

Band Bicep Curl

Band OH Tricep Extension

Band Hammer Curls

Band Skull Crushers

Friday – Legs and Core

Circuit 1 50/10 Repeat for 2 sets

Prisoner Squat

Burpee

Side to Side Lunge

Steam Engine

Circuit 2 50/10 Repeat for 2 sets

Alternating Step Back Lunge

Plank Push Up

Calf Raise Squat

Mountain Climbers

Circuit 3 30/30

Single Leg Deadlift Squat Left

Single Leg Deadlift Squat Right

Russian Twist

Get Ups

Jump Squats

Vups

Circuit 4 20/10 Repeat for 2 sets

Burpee

Speed Squat

Bicycles

Mountain Climbers

Week 2 and Week 4:

Monday – Legs and Shoulders

Circuit 1 50/10 Repeat for 2 sets

Ski Hops

Band Arnold Press

Band Resisted Calf Raise Squats

Band Shoulder Press

Circuit 2 50/10 Repeat for 2 sets

Alternating Walking Lunges

Front Band Raises

Jump Squats

Side Lateral Band Raises

Circuit 3 30/30

Left Leg Side Lunge

Front Band Row

Right Leg Side Lunge

Right Single Arm Shoulder Press

Prisoner Squat

Left Single Arm Shoulder Press

Circuit 4 20/10 Repeat for 2 sets

Speed Squats

Side Lateral Raises

Jump Knee Tucks

Band Military Press

Wednesday - Chest and Back

Circuit 1 50/10 Repeat for 2 sets

Band Resisted Military Push Up

Band Bent Over Row

Reach High/Low Balance Push Up

Band Pull Downs

Circuit 2 50/10 Repeat for 2 sets

Staggered Hand Pushups Left hand forward

Band Pull Out

Staggered Hand Pushups Right hand forward

Band Upright Row

Circuit 3 30/30

Band Resisted Push Up

Band Sumo Deadlift

Fly Push Ups Left

Band Pull Down and Hold last rep for 30 second rest period

Fly Push Ups Right

Band Romanian Deadlift

Circuit 4 20/10 Repeat for 2 sets

Band Pull Down

Band Resisted Wide Push Up

Band Pull Out

Band Resisted Military Push Up

Friday – Arms and Abs

Circuit 1 50/10 Repeat for 2 sets

Alternating Band Bicep Curls

Russian Twist

Overhead Band Tricep Extension

Chair Pose

Circuit 2 50/10 Repeat for 2 sets

Band Iso Hold Bicep Curls

Bicycles

Band Throw the Bomb

Plank Hold

Circuit 3 30/30

Band Congdon Curls

Vups

Band Hammer Curls

Left Oblique Crunch

Band Inside/Outside Bicep Curls

Right Oblique Crunch

Circuit 4 20/10 Repeat for 2 sets

Band Curl up Hammer down

Steam engine

Band Bicep Curls

Mountain Climbers

Conclusion

I hope you have enjoyed this book and found value in the tips, recipes, and workouts from our contributing health and fitness pros, and myself.

Keep at it, don't give up, and work hard for that after picture!

Yours in Health and Fitness,

Kris Crepeau